FIVE BITE DIET

A Review, Analysis, and Beginner's Overview of the Diet Plan

Bruce Ackerberg

mindplusfood

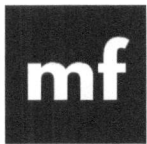

DISCLAIMER

By reading this disclaimer, you are accepting the terms of the disclaimer in full. If you disagree with this disclaimer, please do not read the guide.

All of the content within this guide is provided for informational and educational purposes only, and should not be accepted as independent medical or other professional advice. The author is not a doctor, physician, nurse, mental health provider, or registered nutritionist/dietician. Therefore, using and reading this guide does not establish any form of a physician-patient relationship.

Always consult with a physician or another qualified health provider with any issues or questions you might have regarding any sort of medical condition. Do not ever disregard any qualified professional medical advice or delay seeking that advice because of anything you have read in this guide. The information in this guide is not intended to be any sort of medical advice and should not be used in lieu of any medical advice by a licensed and qualified medical professional.

The information in this guide has been compiled from a variety of known sources. However, the author cannot attest to or guarantee the accuracy of each source and thus should not be held liable for any errors or omissions.

CONTENTS

INTRODUCTION

I want to thank and congratulate you on purchasing this guide.

This guide contains a beginner's overview of the diet, especially its rules, and principles. It also discusses the recommended foods that you should include in your diet as well as foods that you need to avoid. Finally, this guide provides a review and analysis of the pros and cons of this diet. This guide is meant to be a supplemental guide and if you like the overview of what this diet plan entails, you can purchase and read the original work by Dr. Lewis.

More importantly, this guide contains the steps needed to succeed with the Five-Bite Diet. The steps are tailored for beginners like you so that you can easily follow them. They are laid out clearly and are written in detail so that you do not have to dig for more information after you have read this guide.

Before you decide to jumpstart the diet, you need to set your goals. However, you cannot efficiently do so if you do not know your current weight and goal weight. That is why I have included a section in this guide about understanding your normal weight, current weight, and goal weight. It will guide you on how to personalize the program to suit your situation and your needs.

Another important section of this guide is about meal planning. It will help you come up with your very own meal plan where you can take advantage of your creativity to customize each meal and make it more enjoyable.

A section dedicated to providing an objective review of the diet is also included in this guide. The review takes note of the pros and cons of the Five-Bite Diet and provides insights moving forward.

Finally, I have also included some success stories of people who have tried the Five-Bite diet that will keep you inspired and motivated. I also have some important tips to help you focus and stay on track.

Thanks again for purchasing this guide. I hope you enjoy it.

FIVE BITE DIET
OVERVIEW

Brief History

Nowadays, people are more conscious about their health and their looks. Aside from their desire to become fit and healthy, they also want to become slim and sexy. As the number of health buffs grew, many kinds of diet programs have also arisen.

One kind of diet that is gaining popularity these days is the Five-Bite Diet.

This diet was pioneered by Dr. Alwin C. Lewis. He patterned it after the diet of obese and unhealthy individuals who underwent gastric bypass surgery. He noticed how the patients' bodies adapted to the small portions given to them and how they amazingly lost weight. He concluded that eating controlled portions could also work for other people.

He first published a guide about the Five-Bite Diet in 2007 and then he went his way to promote it. The diet rocketed to stardom when it was featured in the Dr. Oz Show, a very popular TV show. Since then, it has gained a lot of followers from around the globe. Today, many are very enthusiastic about it and are eager to try it out.

Diet Rules

The program does not allow for eating breakfast. It is believed that after sleep, the body's metabolism is slow and it needs a little more time to adjust to an additional workload. Hence, food intake in the morning is not suggested. However, drinking coffee, tea, and other sugar-free beverages are permitted. There is no limit as to how much beverage a person drinks, so long as he chooses a low-calorie or calorie-free beverage. It is strongly advised that a diet practitioner drink as much as he can throughout the day to avoid dehydration and prevent his stomach from feeling empty.

The program allows for eating all kinds of food for lunch and dinner. That's right. A diet practitioner can eat any food he or she likes, but portions should be controlled. They are encouraged to eat only five bites of any food per meal. It could be five bites of only one kind of food or a combination of one or more kinds of food. Moreover, a couple of snacks may be taken per day, one snack in the morning and another one in the afternoon. The portions should be controlled as well; only two bites are allowed and nothing more.

The size of a bite varies from person to person. To set a standard measurement, the proponents of the diet suggested that a person's average mouthful is considered equivalent to one bite. All diet enthusiasts should understand that the bite they take must not be too small or too big.

Here is an example of what to eat and how to eat them based on the suggested portions. A morning snack of two bites of apple is enough. Lunch may consist of five bites of pulled pork sandwich or three bites of sirloin steak and two bites of Caesar's salad. Two bites of apple pie or one bite of pizza and one bite of banana would suffice for the afternoon snack. Dinner may consist of three bites of spaghetti, one bite of garlic bread, and one bite of meatballs.

It is always wise for a practitioner to carefully choose healthy and filling foods so that his or her energy can be stretched until the next mealtime. Even if the program is lenient on food choices, he or she must be aware that part of their success greatly depends on what they eat.

Food Suggestions

If a person is used to eating to their stomach's content, eating less will make them hungry now and then. They will have to deal with it smartly by choosing foods that can make their stomach feel full for a longer period. Aside from choosing foods that can curb hunger, they should also look for foods that are packed with vitamins, minerals, and other nutrients. Below are some of the recommended foods:

1. Fruits – If a five-bite diet is on your radar, then turn to fruit for a healthy snack option. Fruits such as apples, oranges, bananas, and berries provide beneficial nutrients and fiber that can help keep you fuller for longer. The best part about these fruits is that they are easily portioned - no need to take up major prep time - just five bites and you're good to go!

2. Vegetables – Eating the right vegetables can be beneficial, as they provide essential vitamins and minerals while helping to manage portion size. Choices like carrots, cauliflower, peppers, spinach, and Brussels sprouts are just some of the many options that could be included in meals. Incorporating these nutrient-dense fruits into meals as part of the five-bite diet can help ensure that individuals get adequate nutrition while also helping them stay within their desired calorie intake.

3. Lean proteins - For those looking to adhere to a five-bite diet, lean proteins such as salmon, chicken breast, and turkey breast are excellent sources of nutritive value. The benefits of these types of protein-rich foods are widely recognized for their muscle growth and overall health-promoting capabilities.

4. Whole grains – When seeking variety for a Five-bite Diet, one of the most important ingredients is whole grains. This nutrient-dense food contains high concentrations of essential vitamins and minerals, such as vitamin B6, iron, and magnesium-- all necessary to support an active lifestyle. Whole grain bread and other products like oats or farro are great choices for incorporating into the diet as they provide sustained energy that can be enjoyed throughout the day.

5. Beans & legumes – Legumes have been shown to provide a variety of nutrients and health benefits when included in the diet. Lentils, chickpeas, and other legumes are excellent sources of protein, dietary fiber, zinc, magnesium, and essential fatty acids. As part of a five-bite diet, they are ideal as they provide these benefits without consuming large amounts of food. Including these healthy legumes in small servings is an easy way to improve overall health on this type of diet plan.

6. Nuts – A five-bite diet is a great way to help those wanting to control their calorie consumption. One component of the five-bite diet is nuts, such as almonds and walnuts. Consuming these nuts offers a satisfying crunch while still allowing individuals to get the benefit of healthy fats. Along with that, they contain protein, zinc, and magnesium – making them a good snack option for anyone needing to watch their intake of calories.

7. Seeds – Eating a handful of sunflower seeds can be an ideal snack when following a five-bite diet. This type of diet is not only beneficial for weight loss but also has considerable health benefits. Sunflower seeds, one of the recommended foods to eat in this diet, are packed with essential vitamins, minerals, and other nutrients

like Vitamin E & B6 and phosphorus, and magnesium. To add extra flavor to your snack experience, incorporate some sesame seeds into the mix.

8. Greek yogurt – Greek yogurt is an ideal choice for those who are following a five-bite diet. Not only does it provide protein, calcium, phosphorus, zinc, and potassium—all essential nutrients —but it also has probiotic properties that can help improve digestion. Plus, the sugar content of Greek yogurt will be kept to a minimum, meaning that you don't have to feel guilty about your healthy snack cravings.

9. Cottage cheese – People on a five-bite diet should make cottage cheese part of their regimen due to its high nutrient content and low caloric value. Since it has high amounts of protein, as well as some essential vitamins and minerals like vitamins A and B complex, iodine, and selenium, cottage cheese is a smart choice for aiding weight loss goals while also offering protection against various illnesses. Additionally, the vitamins and minerals found in this food can help reduce signs of aging, giving health benefits to those who make it part of their diets.

10. Eggs – Eggs are a great choice of food to have on a five-bite diet as they are compact, high in protein and vitamins, and incredibly versatile. Boil them for a quick snack in the morning, scramble them up for dinner, or poach them for lunch - however, if you like to eat them, eggs will provide you with an impressive array of essential nutrients that your body needs. Not just high in protein but ample in omega-3 fatty acids, iron, and vitamins A & B12, there is no reason why eggs should not be included in your diet!

Foods to Avoid

The five-bite diet is an eating plan designed to help people lose weight by reducing their overall calorie intake. It encourages limiting your daily food intake to five bites, or approximately 500 calories. While this type of diet can be effective for some people, it's important to choose the right types of food to make sure you get the most out of it. With that in mind, here are fifteen foods that should be avoided when following a five-bite diet:

1. Fried foods – When it comes to snacks, you want to pick something that won't add to the number of calories you eat in a day and won't make your waistline look larger than it is. However, indulging in fried foods like French fries and onion rings could look like a good idea because they are tasty delights. When you're attempting to limit yourself to just five bits of a meal, the bad fats and salt that are packed into these delectable but unhealthful treats can rapidly build up and make it difficult to stick to your restriction.

2. Red meat – On a five-bite diet, red meats such as hamburgers, steaks, and ribs are optimal foods to avoid. This is because they contain high levels of saturated fat and cholesterol, making them unsuitable for restrictive eating plans.

3. White bread – People who are following the five-bite diet can discover that white bread is not the healthiest option for the meal plans they have created for themselves. Carbohydrates, which are swiftly turned into glucose, which is easily available to the body, can give short-term energy surges, even though the long-term nutritional advantages are essentially nonexistent. These energy surges, on the other hand, may be followed by recurrent feelings of hunger later in the day because just a tiny amount of food is being ingested at any given time.

4. Sugary beverages – Consuming sugary drinks regularly might push you over the daily calorie restriction for a diet like the five-bite plan very fast. There are several popular sodas that each serving has more than 200 calories, even though they offer very few nutrients. Drinking an excessive amount of soda can add pointless calories to your diet, making it more difficult for you to achieve the objectives you have set for yourself. Consider drinking water or unsweetened tea instead of other liquids on a five-bite

diet so that you may keep within the parameters of the eating plan.

5. Processed snacks – Processed snacks such as chips may contain unhealthy fats and oils, artificial flavorings, and preservatives that will not promote a healthier lifestyle. Such choices can derail an individual's weight loss goals and undermine their overall success. Therefore, when it comes to choosing snack options within the five-bite diet plan, opting for fresh fruits or vegetables is recommended to reap nutrition benefits and trackable weight-loss progress.

6. Ice cream – Ice cream is generally considered to be healthy when consumed in moderation; however, if you are following a diet that consists of five bites at a time, you should steer clear of eating it. This is because it contains a large amount of sugar and fat, both of which add considerably to the total calorie count. It is recommended to abstain from having a scoop of ice cream until one is quite certain of the number of bites that are included inside it. If one gives in to further desires, this might throw off their efforts to lose weight.

7. Candy bars – Homemade or store-bought candy bars are not suitable for a five-bite diet because they are full of sugar and often contain unhealthy hydrogenated oils. If consumed regularly, this type of food can quickly lead to obesity and heart disease, so it is important to avoid these items while on the five-bite diet plan.

8. Alcoholic beverages – On the five-bite diet plan, it is important to remember that alcoholic beverages should be avoided due to their high sugar and carb content. With a limited amount of bites allowed, it makes sense to forgo alcoholic drinks altogether since these empty calories don't contribute at all toward sustenance or satisfaction.

9. Fast food burgers & fries – Fried chicken, doughnuts, potato chips, sausages, and other similar items are typically high in carbohydrates, saturated fats, and sodium—all of which

contribute to an unhealthy diet when taken at frequent intervals. For this reason, individuals on a five-bite diet should stay away from these types of food; as they may be more detrimental than beneficial when it comes to maintaining a restricted calorie intake.

10. Doughnuts & pastries – Doughnuts and pastries should be avoided when trying to stick to a five-bite diet because they are high in sugar and calories while offering little nutritional value. These sugary treats often lead to cravings for more sweets or unhealthy snack alternatives. It's best to try and limit sweet treats like doughnuts and pastries if you're attempting a five-bite diet for weight management or overall health purposes.

11. Artificial sweeteners – Many people initially think of artificial sweeteners as being a safe option for snacking since they contain fewer calories than most other snacks. However, over-consumption of these sweeteners can still have adverse effects on one's caloric intake for the day.

12. Processed cheese – Processed cheeses are a food to be avoided when practicing the 5 B's diet, as this method focuses on significantly reducing daily calorie intake. Though tasty, processed cheeses contain a great deal of both saturated fats and sodium, which do not provide any essential vitamins or nutrients. Excessive amounts of fat and salt can quickly send an individual's calorie count past their desired maximum. Thus, an individual should not include processed cheese in their meals while they are attempting to adhere to the 5 B's diet.

13. Snack crackers – Snack crackers are often high in carbs and salt, making them a less desirable option compared to healthier alternatives. Knowing this, it's important to pay attention to how much of them one indulges in as part of their daily food intake as it can quickly add up. Ultimately, for those aiming for a strict caloric deficit, it is best to exclude crackers from the diet altogether.

14. Pie crusts – Due to their trans fat and sodium content, pie crusts and other baked goods should also be avoided to follow the five-bite diet effectively. Pie fillings, while they may seem like a tasty snack option, are not considered a healthy choice due to their high carbohydrates.

15. Salty snacks – Constituting a majority of the average diet, salty snacks like popcorn, pretzels, chips, etc. are consumed far more than is recommended for a healthy lifestyle. High levels of sodium and refined carbohydrates found in most of these snacks make them difficult to work into a five-bite diet to meet daily calorie goals. Therefore, one must be conscious about the selection and preparation of food when incorporating this approach to eating. For these reasons, it is wise to avoid these kinds of salty snacks during a five-bite diet regimen.

HOW TO KICKSTART YOUR DIET

I t is highly recommended that anybody who wishes to try any kind of diet program should make ample preparations first. Before embarking on a diet, he should do his part of the research to gain a better understanding of what he is about to do. This will ensure him a good start with a better success rate.

Here are the things that you must do before you start the diet:

1. Consult with your doctor.
This may sound so cliché for diet beginners. However, it must be understood that this is very important to avoid any potential issues as you continue with the program. You must make sure that your body is capable of handling any effects of the diet. Even if you think that you are healthy enough to go ahead with the program, it still pays to get the green light from a medical expert.

Make sure to consult with your doctor and ask for a routine physical check-up to see if you are fit. If you have any illness or injury, you must be very honest and inform the doctor so that he or she can give you advice and some precautionary measures.

2. Get your BMI.
The body mass index or BMI is a key index that aids in quantifying

a person's tissue mass and it serves as the basis for categorizing an individual as normal weight, underweight, overweight, or obese. To get your BMI, you have to divide your weight in kilograms by your height in meters squared. You can also calculate using your weight in pounds multiplied by 703 and then dividing it by your height in inches squared.

Here is the equation:
BMI = kg/m2 or BMI = (lbs) x (703)/in2

The BMI of individuals who are categorized as normal weight is 18.5 to 25. Underweight individuals have a BMI of below 18.5 while those who are overweight have a BMI of 25 to 30. Those who are obese have a BMI of more than 30.

Shedding some pounds does not always mean you are becoming healthy. You need to get your body mass index so that you will have an idea if there is a need for you to add or lose weight. If you are above the normal weight, it is important that you lose the extra weight without going overboard and subjecting yourself to becoming underweight.

3. Know the normal weight for your height.
You have to be aware that your weight should also be based on your height. If your weight is within the normal and you still feel that you are not fit, maybe you do not need to lose extra weight and what you need is some toning and conditioning of your body.

Here is a guide to help you determine if your weight is within the normal range. If it is more than the normal range, you have to note how much weight you need to lose.

     4' 10" - 91 to 118 lbs.
     4' 11" - 94 to 123 lbs.
     5'   - 97 to 127 lbs.
     5' 1" - 100 to 131 lbs.
     5' 2" - 104 to 135 lbs.
     5' 3" - 107 to 140 lbs.
     5' 4" - 110 to 144 lbs.

```
5' 5"  - 114 to 149 lbs.
5' 6"  - 118 to 154 lbs.
5' 7"  - 121 to 158 lbs.
5' 8"  - 125 to 163 lbs.
5' 9"  - 128 to 168 lbs.
5' 10" - 132 to 173 lbs.
5' 11" - 136 to 178 lbs.
6'     - 140 to 183 lbs.
6' 1"  - 144 to 188 lbs.
6' 2"  - 148 to 193 lbs.
6' 3"  - 152 to 199 lbs.
6' 4"  - 156 to 204 lbs.
```

4. Keep a journal.

Do not underestimate the importance of having a journal while following a diet program. You can jot down notes on it to help you remember valuable information about your diet. It will also help you track your progress and see if you are getting results. It can aid you in making necessary adjustments to your program so that all your efforts will lead to success.

Your journal does not have to be so grand and elaborate. Your journal should contain your current weight, your goal weight, and your timeframe. It should also include detailed information about your meal plan so that you will not be faced with the dilemma of choosing foods at the last minute before the meal. Remember, you are trying to lose weight without causing yourself too much stress.

Daily, you can write down your weight after you wake up in the morning and your weight before you go to bed at night. If this is too much of a hassle for you, you can weigh yourself every week. This is important so that you can check if you are making any progress and if there is a need to make immediate program adjustments.

Include other information that you think is worth noting. It is alright to note down your emotions and your thoughts. Write down your experiences with your food choices and food preparations. Your journal does not only help you keep track of your diet program; it also helps you keep your sanity intact, especially for challenging times when you feel like you cannot continue.

Chocolates and Other Sinful Treats

Many of the meal plans and testimonials to the 5BD mention Snickers bars as a snack, or even breakfast. The additional chocolate in a supposedly low-cal and sugar-free diet may have raised concerns, but just to shed light on this dessert, know that chocolates come from cocoa trees, which is a good source of antioxidants. Dark chocolate, specifically, reduces the risk of heart disease, stabilizes blood sugar, curbs the appetite, and facilitates weight loss.

Chocolate consumption has been linked to lowering the risks of cardiovascular disease. Moreover, Will Clower, a neuroscientist, proved that having A BITE of chocolate and letting it melt on the tongue for 20 minutes sends a signal to the brain that you are full. Whether you eat it alone, or as a dessert to a delicious meal, can delay subsequent snacking. Dr. Lewis wouldn't recommend eating a Snickers bar if it were bad for your physique and metabolism. So grab that Snickers bar, or dark chocolate, and enjoy five bites for a full 20 seconds.

HOW TO MAKE A MEAL PLAN

Y ou can make some tweaks to your meal plan so that your diet will not become boring and monotonous. Since there are not many restrictions as to what you can eat, you should be more creative in mixing and matching food to make each meal an enjoyable one. Happy eating can significantly increase the rate of your success with the diet program.

If you are going to follow the Five-Bite Diet heartily, you will be able to lose fifteen pounds in just seven days. Based on the target weight you want to achieve, you can easily determine how long you need to undergo the diet program. It would be convenient if you can make a complete meal plan for the timeframe that you have set. If your timeframe is just a week or two, a weekly meal plan would do. However, if your timeframe is longer than two weeks, it would be best to do a bi-weekly meal plan and then just repeat it for the next week or two.

Here is a sample of a one-week meal plan:
Monday
Snack: Cheese Omelet
Lunch: Pulled Pork Sandwich
Snack: Banana

Dinner: Grilled Pork and Coleslaw

You can also try cottage cheese instead of a regular one. Cottage cheese is full of protein and calcium. It also helps you feel full longer. No wonder people who add cheese to their daily menu have a more slender frame. You need a little restraint, though, because cheese is also full of fat. Five bites of your favorite cheese would be enough to jumpstart your day or make your omelet more satisfying.

Tuesday
Snack: Oatmeal Pancake
Lunch: Tuna Tortilla Wrap
Snack: Pineapple
Dinner: Baked Salmon and Steamed Green Beans

Now a quick word about eating pineapples for a snack: According to Julie Andrews, a Wisconsin-based chef, pineapples are a great source of fiber, minerals, Vitamin C, manganese, and B vitamins, not to mention that it's got water content that could quickly fill you up. Canned pineapples are a better option but make sure you're not getting those submerged in the syrup. Eat pineapples that are packed in their juices, adds Allison Knott, an NYC dietitian. Consider the syrup a villain, because it will increase your sugar intake. But if you could buy a real pineapple, not the canned, supermarket kind, then that's way better.

Like pineapple, oatmeal is rich in fiber and can fill you for much longer. It also reduces your cholesterol and blood sugar levels. The oatmeal pancake is just one example, but you can vary your oatmeal recipe.

You could add 5 small portions (or bites of apple) or perhaps add grated apples instead. For flavor, add a pinch of cinnamon powder and a tablespoon of natural peanut butter. Enjoying five bites of your oatmeal is now elevated to an enjoyable eating experience.

Wednesday

Snack: Mixed Vegetable Frittata
Lunch: Clubhouse Sandwich
Snack: Yogurt
Dinner: Spaghetti and Greek Salad

Yogurt is a safe bet for a snack, but you can also eat that as a dessert. Again, avoid full-fat and sweet varieties found in most supermarkets. Choose non-fat, or make your own. Dr. Michael Zemel of the University of Tennessee believes that yogurt is effective for maintaining lean muscle mass, which is usually compromised during intermittent fasting.

Nevertheless, including yogurt in your diet amps up your fat-burning mechanism, and fast-tracks your weight loss program. Combining that with 5BD is an effective way to lose a considerable amount of weight.

Thursday
Snack: French Toasts
Lunch: Beef Burger
Snack: Tropical Fruit Salad
Dinner: Seared Tuna and Cucumber Salad

You can have a "skinny" French toast so you are eating something healthy. Instead of white bread, use whole wheat sourdough bread, cinnamon, and nonfat or skimmed milk.

Friday
Snack: Carrot and Hummus
Lunch: Spicy Fried Rice
Snack: Carrot Muffin
Dinner: Fried Chicken and Stir-fried Broccoli

If you noticed, there are two carrot meals in your Friday meal. Carrots have an amazing role in weight loss. The dietary fiber contained in it eases your digestion and ensures regular bowel movement. You could also add carrot juice to your list of beverages (see next chapter). Carrots boost the Vitamin A content in your body and give you your daily dose of antioxidants. They also fight free radicals, prevent the onset of cancerous cells, and effectively beef up your immunity. Because carrots maintain your blood sugar and cholesterol levels, they become a regular staple in anyone's 5BD meal plan.

Saturday
Snack: Deviled Egg
Lunch: Cabbage Rolls
Snack: Baked Sweet Potato
Dinner: Whole-Wheat Rigatoni Pasta and Spring Salad

Compared to ordinary potatoes, sweet potatoes have fewer calories. Consider the latter as the healthier alternative to potatoes (and that includes French fries). Sweet potatoes are also low-glycemic foods that can shrink fat cells, according to a study published in the Journal of Medicinal Food.

Sunday
Snack: Cheesy Stuffed Tomato
Lunch: Pesto Cheese Pizza
Snack: Grilled Cheese Sandwich
Dinner: Quinoa Puttanesca

Quinoa is one of the healthiest foods in the world. It's gluten-free and protein-rich. It is also high in fiber, potassium, vitamin E, magnesium, calcium, and other antioxidants.

Quinoa, a nutritious superfood, contains the flavonoids kaempferol and quercetin, which are also found in cranberries. It improves the body's metabolism and is a better alternative to pasta and bread.

Quinoa is an essential fat-loss ingredient in many 5BD and intermittent fasting meals. Additional benefits of eating quinoa, or adding it to your diet, are healthy teeth and bones, a steady stream of physical energy (no energy crashes!), and reduced cholesterol levels. Eating five bites of quinoa puttanesca can quickly satisfy your hunger.

A 5BD Tracking Sheet

To help you track your first week into the five-bite diet, you can use this simple tracking sheet as a guide. Note: A light breakfast may be included, and the basic 5BD menu has been slightly modified.

Day
Breakfast
Lunch
Dinner
Status (5 bites, overeaten, etc/)

Day 1
Green tea/ black coffee and vitamins
Before lunch: Onion leek, squash, or tomato soup
Protein (beef)
Protein (nuts)

Day 2
Protein, plus vegetables
Protein, plus fruits

Day 3
Repeat day 2, vary the choices

Day 4
Bread (wheat, sugar-free)
Light dessert or pastry

Day 5
Cheese
Protein or milk

Day 6
Protein (fish)
Protein (chicken)

Day 7
Vegetables and fruits
For desserts, drink soda or sparkling water if you like

The example above shows that you can mix and match your meals, and even have a little celebratory meal at the end of the week. The rule is to keep any of your meals to 5 bites.

Here is another sample of a meal plan. Notice how the diet lacks carbohydrates and instead puts more vegetables into the plan. Instead of green tea, the person takes water at the start of his day, then pops in a multivitamin. Green tea is drunk after EACH meal, however. The person opted to not eat pork for personal reasons.

Day
Breakfast
Lunch
Dinner
Status (5 bites, overeaten, etc/)

Day 1
750 ml water and multivitamins
Protein (omelets), green tea
Caesar's salad, green tea

Day 2
Protein (sushi), green tea
Tomatoes, cucumber, and tacos plus green tea

Day 3
Protein (lobster), green tea
Kani salad, green tea

Day 4
Protein (steamed chicken), green tea
Mimosa soup, baked clam, green tea

Day 5

Protein (grilled steak), green tea
Cucumbers, tomatoes, mangoes, green tea

Day 6
Protein (hard-boiled eggs), green tea
Radish, carrots, vinaigrette, green tea

Day 7
Protein (shrimp or grilled chicken)
Buttered and sautéed cauliflowers, green tea

Red wine can be taken in the evenings. A study conducted by Harvard University showed that a glass of red wine daily can reduce the risks of obesity. It also nicked the chances of women gaining weight. Aside from retaining good cholesterol, it reduces the chances of having colon cancer, dementia, and diabetes type 2.

You might read conflicting reports about what to eat in the 5BD. Always remember that the QUALITY of the food is what matters in the five-bite diet. Wine won't have any negative effects on your metabolism if you consume only a glass of it, and in the evenings, when your body is ready to regenerate for the next day.

HOW TO MAKE YOUR BEVERAGES

S ince you will be eating less, the body will tend to lose water weight for the first few days. After that, it will start to lose weight from stored fats. Drinking enough liquid will help sustain your body throughout the program. It will compensate for the lack of solid food in the stomach and make you feel full.

You can settle for just water or you can make it more refreshing and tastier by adding some twists. You can go ahead and make your flavored water because it is preferable to store-bought ones. Commercial flavored water tends to have high sugar content, which is not helpful in weight loss. Another good thing about making your beverage is that you can be sure that your drink also contains nutrients that are beneficial for your health.

For your convenience, you can incorporate flavored water into your meal plan. Make water in different flavors and store them in the refrigerator so that you can drink it anytime and bring it on the go.

Here are 10 of the best-flavored water recipes that you should try:

1. Sassy Minty Water
Combine eight cups of water, one thinly sliced lemon, one thinly

sliced small cucumber, and ten spearmint leaves in a pitcher. Let the flavors blend well by letting it chill in the refrigerator overnight. Strain the water and discard the solid ingredients and then serve.

Mint is known to cure gastrointestinal problems and refresh the palate. Water infused with spearmint, or any beverage with spearmint in it can be beneficial for the heart. Two cups of minty water each day may reduce bad cholesterol levels and triglycerides in your body, not to mention that they are a soothing drink.

2. Herbed Strawberry Water
In a pitcher of water, add two cups of halved strawberries and six basil leaves that have been scrunched. Stir the water well to combine the flavors and then put it in the refrigerator to chill for about two hours.

Strawberries are high in fiber yet low in calories. You can have a strawberry dessert too, or just munch on fruit or two, to boost your weight loss efforts. Teas infused with strawberries help in digestion and make you feel fuller for longer.

3. Classic Apple Cinnamon Water
Rinse one apple, remove the core, and slice it thinly. Add it to a pitcher of water. Add five cinnamon sticks to the water as well. Let it chill in the refrigerator overnight to infuse the flavors. You can adjust the number of cinnamon sticks based on your desired strength of flavor.

Apple cinnamon is also regarded as a detox drink by most people in North America. Many swear by the power of the apple cinnamon drink to eliminate toxins from the body and enrich your system with flavonoids, antioxidants, and vitamin C.

4. Pear Ginger Water
Rinse two pears, remove the cores, and slice them thinly. Put

them in a pitcher filled with 2 liters of water. Add eight thin slices of ginger to the water and stir well. Chill the mixture in the refrigerator for about two hours or longer.

Ginger, like apple cider, is used along with turmeric as a weight-loss drink. Its antioxidant properties help fight free radicals and inflammation. While ginger doesn't directly flush excess fat, it keeps your hunger pangs at bay.

5. Mixed Citrus Water
Place three thin slices of orange, two thin slices of lemon, two thin slices of lime, and three thin slices of grapefruit in a pitcher of water. Stir it well and chill it in the refrigerator for about half an hour before serving.

Citrus water is a popular detox drink and has been known to make up for your hunger pangs. It is low in calories, but can up your energy. Beginning your day with a glass of hot or iced lemon water can kickstart your metabolism and help you burn calories. Besides, lemon water makes your water more exciting to drink!

6. Double Berry Water
Place two cups of blackberries and two cups of raspberries in a pitcher filled with two liters of water. Gently crush berries and stir well to combine. Let the water chill for about an hour or longer.

Just like citrus water, berry water can replace minerals that might be lost while you're on the 5BD. Double berry water makes you healthier, as it refreshes your system, keeps you feeling full, and offers the same nutrients you'll get when you eat the actual fruits.

7. Cucumber Refresher Water
Place five scrunched mint sprigs into a pitcher of water. Add five thin slices of lime and five thin slices of cucumber. Stir well to combine the flavors. Chill the water in the refrigerator overnight and then serve.

Cucumber itself does not significantly make you lose weight, but its water content can keep you feeling fuller. You need lots of water in your body so you don't resort to eating.

8. Tropicana Water
Add two cups of mango chunks and two cups of pineapple chunks into a pitcher of water. You can also add one thin slice of lemon or lime to bring out the sweetness of the fruits. Chill the water for about two hours and then serve.

Moreover, Tropicana water burns fat quickly and provides you with the fiber you need to better digest your food.

9. Spiced Chia Water
Add one thinly sliced orange, two tablespoons of chia seeds, three cinnamon sticks, and half a teaspoon of maple syrup. Stir well to combine all the flavors. Chill the water overnight in the refrigerator before serving.

If you're concerned about chia seeds supplies, don't worry. It's fast becoming a staple in weight loss diets. Chia seeds are believed to curb your appetite because they are rich in fiber. Eating 30 g of chia seeds daily can help you lose weight, although spiced chia water will do.

10. Kiwi Water
Combine eight cups of water, three scrunched mint sprigs, one thinly sliced kiwi, three thin slices of ginger, and half a tablespoon of honey. Place the water in the refrigerator and chill for two hours or more before serving.

But kiwi water isn't the only beverage you can make out of this super fruit. You can also get your hands on a kiwi smoothie. Kiwi, a good source of Vitamins E, K, and C, potassium, and folate, is known to improve digestion and boost metabolism. The enzyme actinidin helps break down proteins (perfect for your protein-rich diet) and breaks down fat molecules.

To make your kiwi smoothie, prepare diced kiwi, yogurt, almonds, and honey. You can add spearmint to taste. There is no need to be afraid of the calories and sugar in yogurt – choose sugar-free ones in the supermarket, or create your yummy Greek yogurt.

HOW TO MAKE
THE DIET WORK

The average calorie intake of an adult is about 2,500 calories. Calories that are not burned by the body will be stored as fats. Slow metabolism and a sedentary lifestyle are some of the reasons why calories are not burned. If a person eats a lot of food, it can also mean that he is consuming a lot of calories. High-calorie consumption will likely lead to weight gain.

Controlled portion intake would mean less calorie intake. Even if a person takes large bites, he may consume only 800 calories or fewer in a day. With lesser calories, his body will spend less time burning them and will spend more time burning the stored fats. Low-calorie intake will eventually lead to weight loss.

Here are things that you should do to make the diet work for you.

1. Be responsible.
The Five-Bite Diet program teaches you to be responsible for controlling your portion for you to obtain positive results. So, take responsibility and stick with it.

The program is very easy to follow because you will not be bothered to count calories. Having the freedom to eat anything you want while dieting is a less stressful way to lose weight. When you enjoy what you are doing, you will tend to follow through with what you have started; hence, you are already partly assured that you will hit your goal.

However, you should be very cautious with what you are doing because your body will need some time to adjust to the sudden change in calorie intake. Your metabolism might be slowed down and your immune system's resistance may be decreased. You may experience side effects, which include nausea, heart palpitations, and headache.

2. Take supplements.
To help your body stay on track and keep your health from being derailed, you need to make sure that you take supplements daily so that you can still keep your vitamin and minerals level optimized even if you are on a diet.

An important mineral to supplement your diet is sodium. Low sodium levels may make the body dehydrated and lethargic. Good sources of sodium are Himalayan salt and another fortified table salt. However, you must avoid too much salt consumption because it can make your body retain more water. High water retention could lead to more weight gain.

In choosing mineral supplements, choose the ones that contain ample amounts of potassium and calcium. Low levels of potassium can affect muscular functions and can make you sluggish. Low calcium can lead to bone loss. Other minerals to look for in a supplement are iron, magnesium, and phosphorus.

Regarding vitamin supplements, you can choose multivitamins so that you can get most of the vitamins that you need. Important vitamins to be optimized during your diet are the B complex vitamins such as vitamins B1, B2, B6, and B12. They help the body maintain normal body processes. Vitamin C is also essential to help your body fight infections.

Lastly, do not cut back on fats. Your body needs good fats to keep your body processes functioning well. Be discriminated against with your preference, though. What you need are healthy fats or unsaturated fats. Good sources of unsaturated fats oils such as coconut oil and olive oil. They contain fatty acids that can help the body speed up its metabolism and boost your body to burn more calories.

3. Stop cravings.
There will be days that you may feel that you are starving but you should not let it destroy your focus. Convince your mind that you are not actually hungry, that you are just bored and you just want to eat something. Instead of thinking about eating, drink water instead. Eventually, your mind will learn the difference between hunger and boredom.

Nevertheless, food cravings can be indications also that your body is lacking certain minerals. Instead of giving in, take it as a call to make adjustments in your meal plan and try to incorporate alternative foods to make up for the lacking nutrients.

If you crave pasta, bread, and other carbohydrate-rich foods, it means you need to replenish nitrogen. Add meats, beans, nuts, and seeds to your diet.

If you crave salty foods, it means your silicon and choline levels are low. Add nuts, seeds, and fish to your diet.

If you crave oily foods, it means your calcium level is depleting. Add more green leafy vegetables, milk, and other dairy products to your diet.

If you crave chocolates, it means your magnesium level is low. Add more fruits, vegetables, and nuts to your diet.

If you crave sweets, it means several minerals such as phosphorus, tryptophan, and chromium need to be supplemented. Add cruciferous vegetables, eggs, poultry, as well as whole grains to your diet.

SUCCESS STORIES AND TIPS

Even if many people call the five-bite diet a fad diet, it is still sweeping the world because many can swear by its effectiveness in weight loss. Well-known personalities and celebrities are also joining the bandwagon. A prominent individual who is very vocal about his success with the diet program is Gregory Mantell, a seasoned TV producer, anchor, and reporter. He is also the host of a popular online talk show.

Mr. Mantell said that he needed to lose weight and stay in great shape because of the nature of his job. Like other diet enthusiasts, he had also tried several diet regimens before doing the Five-Bite Diet. His previous dieting experiences were all failures and he ended up frustrated with his situation.

When he came across the Five-Bite Diet, he felt the urge to try it and he was in for a great surprise. After practicing the diet for a couple of weeks, he lost a total of twenty pounds. He was so overwhelmed by the results. He said that he was motivated and believed that he could continue to lose more weight. He was so certain that he could do the diet program for the long term.

Aside from him, other individuals experienced positive results and many of them are now talking about their success and sharing them through social media. Many of those who had succeeded can be seen joining online forums and helping other diet enthusiasts succeed as well. Some of them have even made the extra effort to increase their online presence by doing videos and interactive sites so they can reach out and guide other people.

Here are some tips from people who have succeeded:

1. Find a support group.
A diet that lets you eat anything you want is indeed very easy to follow. However, not all days are easy and there will be days when you may face a lot of obstacles. Having people who understand you and what you are doing is a great way to keep yourself motivated and stay on track. Look for online forums and join the one that you feel you are more comfortable with.

2. Inform your family and friends.
It can be difficult to hold yourself back from eating if you see people around you eating their hearts out. Let people who are close to you know what you are up to and ask them to help you out. If they become aware of your diet plans and they give you support, your everyday eating will be less stressful.

3. Set an eating pattern.
Based on your daily schedules and routines, identify the perfect time to eat your meals and snacks. Be sure to eat at the exact time every day so that your body's metabolism can create a rhythm and get comfortable with it. Do not be discouraged if you cannot create a pattern soon enough. It is going to be a gradual process and it may take a few days before your body can get the hang of it.

4. Extend your patience.
The body's reaction to the diet varies from person to person. If you feel that you have a hard time progressing with the program, give yourself more time. You have the power over your time, the same way you have power over your portion. Positive results do not come to those who easily give up.

5. Reward yourself.

Treat yourself at the end of the program. Whatever the result of your diet is, you must make sure to thank and congratulate yourself. Just remember not to treat yourself to food. Otherwise, you will only put on more weight. You may treat yourself to a spa or you can go shopping for smaller clothes. Do anything that will make you feel pampered and relaxed.

Some Personal Observations

You can drink as much of anything as long as it doesn't contain calories. Water, hence, is your best friend. Diet soda is OK, although most people on a five-bite diet would rather keep it healthy. Diet soda may still spike your sugar up.

Some people on a diet advice drinking a cup of black coffee, paired with a multivitamin, just to keep the hunger pangs at bay. They have observed that the body goes into a fast mode in the evening and does not crave food until mid-morning.

A Total Change of Lifestyle

The five-bite diet is a total overhaul of your lifestyle for some. While other dieters think of it as the quickest way to lose weight, others have chosen to adopt the five-bite diet and maintain their weight and figure. The body's only source of energy is sugar, so this must be converted right away into fuel. The body only needs five bites of glucose sugar to work. Anything beyond that is stored as fat. The objective of the five-bite diet is to transform the body into a fat-burning machine.

Once you see the logic behind the five-bite diet, you'll understand why some dieters would rather make it part of their lifestyle forever. The five-bite diet keeps you disciplined, as in the case of Shannon. It helps you train your mind to eat a certain amount of food. Eating must not be so much physical activity as it is a mental activity.

Is this what the French call a portion-control diet?

The answer is YES. The five-bite diet tells you to eat with your brains, not with your tummy. It trains you to eat not when you're hungry, but when it's time to eat. Similarly, you stop eating because you're not hungry anymore. You don't wait until you are full. Suffice it to say, the five-bite diet doesn't want you to go on a hunger strike. On the contrary, it encourages you to eat balanced meals.

Let Your Stomach Calibrate

Hunger is a mental phenomenon. Because your body is conditioned to eat every 2 hours, it tends to send you hunger signals when you still haven't eaten at the given time. In the same manner, if your body is used to eating A LOT, it will look for that amount of food each day. Eating mindlessly adds to the problem because you'll simply keep popping food into your mouth.

This is precisely the reason why people on portion control or 5BD have to do NOTHING ELSE while they eat. Eating must not be a distraction; it should be a mindful and pleasurable experience, meant to be savored. Moreover, dieters are advised to enjoy every morsel. Yes, make those five bites worth your time so they would be more attuned to the taste of what they are eating.

When you pay attention to your food, you also enjoy its flavors. Chewing slowly also makes up for the 5 bites that you need to satiate your stomach with. After doing this consistently for 4 days, you'll notice that your stomach has recalibrated. Do so for about 2 weeks, then include more variety into your food.

You often see 5BD testimonials and tutorials telling you to eat 2 oz of Snickers. You might think that's a rule that everybody must follow. But Snickers isn't necessary. It's just the ideal and probably the most popular example of a chocolate snack. Nevertheless, any dessert is OK as long as you keep it to 5 bites, nothing more and nothing less.

Five Bites of Everything Doesn't Mean Five Huge Bites

A silly question that goes around the Net these days is that if you ate a Big Mac in five bites, would you still lose weight?

People seem to be missing the point of 5BD. This diet starts right in the preparation of your meals. The quality of what you eat is significant to losing weight as well. The Big Mac theory already presents two problems.

One, it's junk food. Five bites of junk won't give you anything but extra fat and calories. Think of the salt! Think of the meat extenders that you're feeding your body with. Your body is not even worth 5 bites of junk.

You might argue that chocolate bars such as Snickers are considered junk food. This is where we analyze the next problem: size.

So you were told to eat only five bites, right? But what you are forgetting is the size of each bite. Again, Dr. Lewis advises you to not go beyond one swallow. A small bite compared to a large bite makes all the difference. Not because you ate 5 huge bites of Big Mac means you are losing weight. That's not mindful and healthy eating.

Now, what if you get suddenly hungry and you're still on Day 1?

It takes 3 days for the body to get adjusted to your new diet. Days 1 to 3 are your litmus tests. You need loads of self-control to get past them and not backslide into your old diet. Other people had to wait for a week or two before they were able to adjust to what they were eating.

The key is to vary your meals, keep a diary of what you eat, and simply stay steadfast with your weight loss goals. Avoid going to the bathroom to check your scale. This only puts you in an anticipatory mood and you might feel disappointed if you don't see results right away. The earliest time that you should be checking your weight should be after two weeks. By then you would have recalibrated your stomach and food intake.

Know that hunger is purely psychological. You were accustomed to eating like a rabbit eats its veggies, so naturally, your body will crave this activity. If you still feel hungry on the third day, distract yourself. Start moving around. Take your mind off your body.

Another way is to drink water. Water fills the body and cheats the mind that it's already full, even if it isn't. Iced green tea, the sugar-free kind, also curbs false hunger. Green tea has weight loss properties, too, so you're hitting two birds with one stone here!

Can you simply eat what you like and burn calories through exercise?

Weight loss has something to do with a diet more than exercise. If your goal is to pack on the pounds or lose extra fat, cardio exercises would do you well. But if you are just starting on the weight loss journey, it is wise to spend the FIRST 3 days on the 5BD.

The logic behind most diets is this: weight loss is 20 percent exercise and 80 percent diet. If you exercise for an hour and sweat a lot, yet eat a calorie-packed chocolate cake in one go, you have defeated the purpose of your exercise.

According to Dr. Lewis, exercise keeps your head in the game. It aids your weight loss by helping you shed up to 20 pounds in two weeks. But if you also jumpstart on the 5BD, you'll lose more than you expect.

You must forgo your exercise for the first 3 days of 5BD. Give your body some allowance to adjust. Should you incorporate exercise, keep it to a minimum.

Walking is the safest yet most effective form of exercise. It greatly complements the 5BD and does not strain your muscles. Whether it's a brisk walk to the market or a leisurely walk in the park, you'll feel good about your body in no time. Walking as a meditative activity is a plus.

You'll be surprised that not everybody who's in the 5BD is into exercise. And they still lose weight.

Is there a modified version of the 5BD?

The 5BD can be modified to suit your body. The reason most fad diets don't work is that doctors and nutritionists present these diets in a one-size-fits-all approach. Each body is different. It has a different shape and genetic makeup. Your weight can also be influenced by several factors, not just food and exercise. Genetics and lifestyles can be a deterrent to your weight loss program. Thus, diets such as 5BD are modified and personalized.

Can you limit the calories in the 5BD Diet?
The body can burn more calories if you're able to meet its caloric requirements – nothing more and nothing less. This is why eating protein first thing in the morning is ideal, and why superfoods can make a tremendous change in your body.

Eating apples is another trick that five-bite dieters suggest. Apples help you feel fuller, suppress your appetite, and stabilize your blood sugar levels. Taking five bites of an apple before your dinner can help you absorb fewer calories.

PROS & CONS OF THE FIVE-BITE DIET

I ndeed, the 2007 guide Why Weight Around? written by Dr. Alwin C. Lewis took the world by storm as it rose to become a household name for weight-loss programs. After reading all about it and how you can succeed by following the program as well as several success stories, it's still worth remembering that the Five-Bite Diet had its flaws.

To carefully and intelligently consider committing to this program, you need to learn first about its advantages and disadvantages. Below are some of them for you to consider:

Pros

It works – One of the best parts of the Five-Bite Diet is that it teaches practitioners to control the portion of calorie intake, which is a tried and tested strategy in successful weight loss programs throughout the globe because it's not as restrictive. Unlike many diet regimes, the Five-Bite Diet does not place restrictions on the type of food you can eat. The type of food you eat is hardly considered at all.

The main focus is the portion you take per meal and per day.

This works because it helps avoid feelings of deprivation that usually comes with diet programs that restrict food intake among practitioners. As a result, you're not likely to resort to binge eating due to feelings of deprivation.

It's easy to follow – This diet does not require you to maintain a complex food list, do constant calculations, or keep track of every little thing you eat. All you have to do is not eat more than five bites. It's not rocket science.

Reduces joint pain and risk of diabetes. According to a study conducted by Dr. Rena R. Wing and Wei Lang in 2011, modern weight-loss approaches such as the five-bite diet can reduce joint pain and chances of getting type 2 diabetes. Weight change and improvements had a significant correlation, especially because there was better glycemic control. This further emphasizes the importance of eating healthy food, even when you're already into the 5BD. It is far better to eat five bites of quality meals than five bites of junk food.

Reduces the time you need to exercise. While nobody's stopping you from hitting the gym, you certainly need not sweat it all out. Since you have control over your calories, you can burn them with little movement. It's also not advisable to spend hours in the gym when you're on the 5BD, because you may not have the energy to do so.

It liberates you from calorie counting. Now isn't that fun? You don't need to monitor your calories because you have control over how much you consume. You can also stop checking the nutritional information on the back of food and beverage packages.

Cons

A five-bite diet is a restrictive eating plan that involves consuming only five bites of food per day. While this type of diet may help some people achieve their weight loss goals, there are also many disadvantages associated with it.

The first drawback is that it is very difficult to adhere to because of how limiting it is. If you just eat five bits of food, you will not get the essential number of calories or nutrients for proper nourishment, which might cause you to feel tired and weak. Even if you are successful in sticking to this regimen, your body will still be missing out on essential vitamins and minerals, which in the long term might cause a wide variety of health issues.

The second disadvantage is that the potential benefits of this diet cannot be sustained in the long term. Since it restricts food intake so much, once you go off the plan, you may find yourself gaining back any weight that was lost. This means that you may end up needing to start over again if you want to see any lasting results from your efforts.

The third disadvantage is that it leads to an unhealthy relationship with food. Eating such small amounts on such a strict schedule can cause psychological distress as well as feelings of deprivation which can have serious negative impacts on mental health over time. Furthermore, since the five-bite diet does not involve counting calories or tracking macronutrient intake, this could lead to a lack of awareness about what types of foods are healthy for a person's body and lifestyle.

Fourthly, individuals who practice five-bite diets also risk nutritional deficiencies as they are not receiving enough micronutrients from their limited daily meals. Inadequate amounts of certain vitamins such as Vitamin A and folate can have serious implications on one's health in addition to leading to poor digestion, immune system dysfunction, and other potential issues related to inadequate nutrition.

Fifthly, since there are no guidelines on what should be eaten in each bite, individuals may be tempted to pick unhealthy snacks or processed foods instead of balanced meals with an emphasis on fruits and vegetables due to their convenience or enjoyable taste sensation—further adding fuel to existing health risks already posed by the restricted caloric intake itself as outlined previously hereinabove.

Sixthly, there is little room for errors while practicing five-bite diets due to its extreme nature–one slip-up could result in increased calorie intake beyond desirable levels while triggering further cravings–making adherence even more challenging than initially assumed via thought experiments before engaging in this restrictive eating protocol regime.

Seventhly, following the five-bite diet increases an individual's chances of developing an eating disorder due to its extreme restrictions which can create intense cravings for foods typically prohibited under its regimes together with strong feelings of guilt bordering shame after every "mistake". Similarly, it also increases one's tendency towards weighing themselves obsessively as well as scrutinizing their bodies closely leading down paths associated with various disordered eating behaviors such as binging & purging syndrome.

Ultimately, when it comes to dietary habits, removing all of a person's particular food preferences by prohibiting any kind of treats or guilty pleasure might, in the end, only make the situation worse. Cutting away all of the delicious foods that a person adores can cause mental tension and unhappiness, which can have a bad effect on their adherence rate before they have ever had the opportunity to begin working toward their weight reduction objectives efficiently.

The benefits of applying this approach must exceed the problems of the five-bite diet, even though the five-bite diet does have certain limitations. Users can regain control over the amount of food they consume and have less anxiety at meal times if they restrict themselves to consuming only five bits of food each day and remove harmful sources of temptation from their environment. This has the potential to be a significant role in assisting with the accomplishment of desired goals.

CONCLUSION

Anyone serious about losing weight needs to understand that weight loss is not an overnight phenomenon. It takes a great deal of determination and perseverance to finish a program successfully. The same is true for the Five-Bite Diet. Without the foundational goals you set at the beginning of the program, you will most likely fail.

On the other hand, success stories have described in detail how this plan, if implemented correctly, can do wonders for your body and self-esteem. Losing those unwanted pounds can be a walk in the park if you strictly follow the instructions laid out in this guide. The diet plan also mentions that exercise is an important aspect of the overall success of the program. Make it a point to jog in the morning if you can and burn off some of those calories. The endorphin rush will make you feel good too. Also, don't forget to take your multivitamin supplements.

While it is an effective crash course diet, the Five-Bite Diet is not a perfect program. In the previous chapter, you have learned some of its advantages as well as its disadvantages notably the program's long-term consequences. Please take note that this is not meant to scare you or discourage you from going through the diet regime. Instead, it is meant to encourage you to think critically about what you can do to lose weight.

The road to weight loss (and eventually, a healthy lifestyle) is long and winding. Make sure to pack all of the grit, determination, and sheer motivation you can as you begin your journey to a healthier you.

Thank you again for purchasing this guide.

If you enjoyed this guide, please take the time to share your thoughts and post a review. It would be greatly appreciated.

REFERENCES AND HELPFUL LINKS

How does the five bite diet work? (n.d.). Healthy Eating | SF Gate. Retrieved March 2, 2023, from https://healthyeating.sfgate.com/five-bite-diet-work-9698.html.

I tried the five bite diet because I thought there was nothing worse … (n.d.). Retrieved March 2, 2023, from https://www.bodyandsoul.com.au/diet/i-tried-the-five-bite-diet-because-i-thought-there-was-nothing-worse-than-counting-calories-i-was-wrong/news-story/21d04f8ff0a32a5f1c859fb69d37459c.

Nast, C. (2010, February 11). Have you heard of the "five bite" diet? Glamour. https://www.glamour.com/story/have-you-heard-of-the-five-bit.

The 5 bite diet review: Does it work for weight loss? (2019, July 2). Healthline. https://www.healthline.com/nutrition/5-bite-diet.

This "5 bite diet" is all you need to shed kilos in week! (n.d.). ANI News. Retrieved March 2, 2023, from https://www.aninews.in/news/lifestyle/fitness/this-5-bite-diet-is-all-you-need-to-shed-kilos-in-week20190703070046/.

World, D. (2014, December 28). 5 bite diet plan by dr. Alwin lewis. Disabled World. https://www.disabled-world.com/fitness/diets/5-bite.php.